RUNAWAY MEDICINE

What You Don't Know May Kill You

CAROLYN BARBER, M.D.

All rights reserved: This book or parts thereof may not be reproduced in any form, stored in any retrieval system, or transmitted in any form by any. means— electronic, mechanical, photocopy, recording, or otherwise— without prior written permission of the publisher, except as provided by United States of America copyright law or for brief examples in a review.

Disclaimer: This book by Carolyn Barber or parts thereof are intended to provide only a general guide on this subject matter. Neither the author nor the publisher provides any legal, medical or professional advice. This book does not provide complete information on the subject matter covered. While the author has undertaken diligent efforts to ensure accuracy, there is no guarantee of accuracy or of no errors, omissions, or typographical errors. The author and publisher shall have no liability or responsibility to any person or entity and hereby disclaim all liability, including without limitation, liability for consequential damages regarding any claim, loss or damage that may be incurred, or alleged to have been incurred, directly or indirectly, arising out of information provided in this book or in any supplementary material.

Acknowledgement: I would like to thank my editor, Mark Kreidler, for his guidance and collaboration, and for encouraging me in this endeavor.

Copyright © 2020 Carolyn Barber, MD
Published 2020
Printed in the USA on recycled acid-free paper
ISBN: 978-0-578-23672-8

I was a 23-year-old investment banker, working ludicrous hours in New York and training for marathons on the side, when cancer first entered my life. In the three decades since, the disease has not been a constant companion, but certainly a ride-along. It was not always speaking loudly, but it was back there somewhere.

Now that there is a possibility that my cancer is back, questions about some of the decisions that my doctors and I made in 1987 have resurfaced.

Was my radiation really necessary? Could we have more thoroughly discussed the poor base of research related to my type of cancer, and would knowing more about the uncertainties and potential long-term complications have made a difference in my choices?

Is the way we treated my cancer back then the reason I'm still here 30 years later, or is it possibly the cause of the new nodules discovered in my neck? Perhaps it is a combination of both?

There were so many questions I did not know to ask when, standing at a pay phone on the East Side of Manhattan, I heard a voice at the other end from Texas tell me that the initial pathology report had been incorrect. Rather than a benign growth, I had a malignant tumor in my mouth.

I know more now. I want you to know more, too.

On a daily basis in the U.S., unnecessary medical tests, treatments and surgeries actively harm patients at astounding rates. Physicians fail to adequately inform subjects about the downstream risk of procedures. The pharmaceutical and biomedical industry influence doctors' decision-making, actively bias major product research, pay key players to grease the skids for expanded sales, and fail to disclose the harm some of their medicines and devices can do.

Patients, many of them vulnerable and afraid, are suggestible in the extreme, often not understanding all the factors at play. By the time they realize that one ill-fated decision may lead to more and more medical intervention and cost, it's often too late.

This is by no means a full picture of the healthcare industry, but it may be the piece that is the least well understood. In my case, I likely would have come to many of these conclusions on my own, by experiencing, replaying and evaluating the key sequences and decisions specific to my care — hard-won knowledge from 30 years spent living with a disease.

But I will never have to test that theory, because I have seen it all first-hand already. From the other side of the gurney.

Not long after I began my work as an Emergency Department physician, a few years after my own diagnosis, the ER director singled me out as the department's "top income generator on a per-hour basis," a designation that I was not aware existed. He said he wanted to know my secret.

My secret: I was inexperienced and afraid of missing something, so I was ordering too many tests and likely hospitalizing too many patients. But my boss wasn't complaining.

It is important to know, as a healthcare consumer in America, that you are far more likely to be steered toward tests and procedures than away from them, even if those interventions don't have a proven clinical benefit. In fact, a *USA Today* analysis of medical databases and government records found that 10% to 20% of all surgeries in certain specialties are likely unnecessary.[1] It is estimated that such unnecessary testing and surgeries add up to more than $200 billion in extra spending per year, according to the Institute of Medicine.[2]

---

[1] Peter Eisler & Barbara Hansen, "Doctors perform thousands of unnecessary surgeries," *USA Today*, June 20, 2013.
https://www.usatoday.com/story/news/nation/2013/06/18/unnecessary-surgery-usa-today-investigation/2435009/
[2] Mark Smith, MD." Best Care at Lower Cost. Institute of Medicine Committee on the Learning Health Care System in American." *The National Academies of Sciences 2013.*

These procedures come at tremendous human cost.[3] At least 30,000 deaths in the U.S. each year are linked to mistakes and injuries caused by superfluous medical treatment. Some sources even put the number at double that. A survey by the Department of Health and Human Services, meanwhile, found that one in eight Medicare patients was actively harmed by medical treatment *while hospitalized*. Nearly half of those cases, HHS said, were preventable.[4] Incredibly, the equivalent of ten jumbo planes crashing is the estimated number of people who die every week in the U.S. due to avoidable medical error.[5]

As physicians, we are trained to be proactive. We don't want to miss anything. As a matter of behavior, both innate and learned, we are not particularly good at doing less. Such has been my experience, but that only represents one side of the mirror.

That's why we wind up overprescribing and overtreating you on such a massive, continuous scale. Incredibly, with a population of 325 million people in the U.S., we order approximately 15 million

---

[3] "Unnecessary Medical Tests," *Healthcarefinancenews.com*, May 24, 2017, https://www.healthcarefinancenews.com/news/unnecessary-medical-tests-treatments-cost-200-billion-annually-cause-harm

[4] Levinson DR *"Adverse Events in Hospitals: National Incidence among Medicare Beneficiaries"*, US Dept of Health and Human Services, https://psnet.ahrq.gov/issue/adverse-events-hospitals-national-incidence-among-medicare-beneficiaries

[5] Sarah Kliff, *"8 Facts That Explain What's Wrong with American Health Care"*, vox.com, etc Jan 20, 2015 https://www.vox.com/2014/9/2/6089693/health-care-facts-whats-wrong-american-insurance

nuclear imaging studies, 100 million MRIs and CT scans, and close to 10 billion blood tests on patients every year.[6] We're not talking about a little pinch of "err on the side of caution" — we are talking about runaway medicine with patients on board a system with no brakes, few guardrails, and no one fully at the controls.

And there are other forces at play in this healthcare equation that you, as a patient, must reckon with as well. The problem is, no one much wants to tell you about them — especially not Big Pharma or the medical device industry, which loom so large in this conversation.

Our healthcare system is in desperate need of a checkup. Here is a perspective from my colleagues' ranks: In a large-scale survey in 2017, doctors from the American Medical Association (AMA) said that nearly a quarter of all the tests they performed were unnecessary, along with more than 20 percent of the prescriptions they wrote.[7] Every tenth surgical procedure, they said, didn't need to be done. The most commonly cited explanation for this was the fear of getting sued, and there is no question that is a genuine worry. In fact, a very large study found that specialty physicians

---

[6] Atul Gawande, "Overkill," *The New Yorker*, May 11, 2015
https://www.newyorker.com/magazine/2015/05/11/overkill-atul-gawande
[7] Heather Lyu, "Overtreatment in the United States", NCBI, PLOS One, Sept 6, 1917,
https://www.ncbi.nlm.nih.gov/pmc/articles/PMC5587107/#!po=73.5294

with a financial interest in an on-site lab facility were eight times more likely to order common lab tests than physician non-owners. Beyond that, more than 70 percent of the survey respondents said they believed doctors were more likely to perform unnecessary procedures when they profited from them.[8] That is the fee-for-service model of healthcare compensation at work, magnified by the commercial influence of pharmaceutical and device manufacturers.

I neither knew nor thought about any of this when I was diagnosed at the age of 23; I wanted help. The tumor on the roof of my mouth had grown, gradually but persistently, until it was the size of a golf ball. It bled on my pillow at night. After initial care back home in Texas, doctors at Sloan Kettering Cancer Center ran more tests that confirmed their suspicion: I had a rare form of salivary gland cancer, and the tumor itself was sitting atop a large artery. It was delicate and dangerous, and it would take two surgeries to get it all.

What followed led me to my current life path. Inspired by the care and skill of my surgical oncologist and the support I received during my recovery, I left banking, took pre-med classes, entered

---

[8] Tara Bishop, "Laboratory Test Ordering at Physician Offices with and without On-Site Laboratories", *J Gen Intern Med.* 2010 Oct; 25(10): 1057–1063. https://www.ncbi.nlm.nih.gov/pmc/articles/PMC2955467/

the Johns Hopkins School of Medicine, and completed a residency at Stanford University Hospital. I have spent the last 25 years caring for patients in the emergency departments of several teaching hospitals. It has been an absolute privilege and a meaningful way for me to give back.

But there was another component to my care back then. With little discussion beforehand, I was scheduled for and underwent radiation therapy as a complementary treatment to my surgeries. My radiation oncologist briefed me on a few of the potential short-term effects of such treatments. I might experience a dry mouth, for example, or lose hair, or develop some blisters on my skin.

The potential long-term risks? Not so much.

Some complications from the treatment changed my daily life forever. Even a minor wound in the irradiated area can be very slow to heal. More significantly, a procedure to close a small hole on the roof of my mouth by using a skin flap failed immediately, very likely because of the prior radiation. The hole became much larger, and it now affects my speech to the point that I am often misunderstood, especially on the phone. I experience chronic sinusitis with fairly frequent acute infections. Recently, and for the first time, I developed a serious blood infection originating from my sinuses that knocked me flat for three days and resulted in an early departure home from overseas.

Radiation may well have been the right call at the time; we didn't have a lot to go on, as my diagnosis was unusual. More information on such operations and multimodal treatment regimens is available now, including potential long-term issues and, for some, very low rates of effectiveness. They continue to be advocated in the National Comprehensive Cancer Network guidelines. Yet my reading of the literature shows little evidence of any treatment-related survival benefit for patients, and randomized clinical trials (our gold standard) are virtually nonexistent for my tumor.[9] For me, if I undertake expensive treatments with dangerous side effects, I want to know they have a good chance of meaningfully prolonging my life.

Such treatments offer patients hope and provide them choices. Significantly, they also make money. They make money for the drug or device manufacturer, for the hospital or medical center, and often for the physician. Many other factors may swing into view here, and I'll address them in a moment, but the money looms large.

---

[9] Young Kwang Chae, Adenoid cystic carcinoma: current therapy and potential therapeutic advances based on genomic profiling, *Oncotarget*. Nov 10 2015; 6(35): 37117–37134. Published online 2015 Aug 21.
https://www.ncbi.nlm.nih.gov/pmc/articles/PMC4741919/

If you're an average adult, there's a reasonable chance you know someone who has had a cardiac stent implanted to fight coronary disease. In the U.S., we place such stents in about 100,000 patients each year who have stable heart disease, at a cost of roughly $25,000 to $28,000 per procedure. We do this despite high-quality scientific studies showing that stents neither save more lives, nor reduce the chances of patients having a heart attack than simply taking heart medicine.[10] A massive global study in 2019 called the ISCHEMIA Trial, came to the same conclusion.[11] A person with stable heart disease, the study said, might be just as well off making some lifestyle changes and taking something as basic as aspirin.

Researchers at Stanford examined data from more than 900,000 privately insured patients who had experienced chest pain but lacked clear signs of heart disease. The study found that those who underwent more testing (versus those who were tested less) had higher rates of cardiac catheterizations, angioplasties, and even cardiac surgeries.

These downstream procedures cost money, but ultimately made

---

[10] William Boden, "Optimal Medical Therapy with or without PCI for Stable Coronary Disease, *NEJM*, April 12, 2007
https://www.nejm.org/doi/full/10.1056/NEJMoa070829
[11] Judith Hochman, "Ischemia Trial" *JAMA*, Feb 27, 2019,
https://jamanetwork.com/journals/jamacardiology/fullarticle/2725865

no difference in later admissions for heart attacks.[12] More testing led to more procedures with more risk — but to no appreciable end, suggesting routine testing might not be warranted.

Spinal fusion? It's a $40 billion annual industry, making it the most popular elective surgery in the U.S. and major component of a $100 billion yearly intake on back-related surgeries alone. It also seldom works: multiple studies show it to be no more effective than nonoperative treatment such as physical therapy and exercise, in patients with chronic low back pain.[13] Yet the frequency of spinal fusion surgeries, at a current price tag above $80,000, skyrocketed by 600 percent over a 20-year period beginning in the 1990s.[14]

Discectomies, popular procedures for those with herniated discs, have repeatedly been proved no more effective over the long term than having no surgery at all. Perhaps more concerning, the rate of complications from these back surgeries runs as high as 18 to

---

[12] Alexander Sandhu, " Cardiovascular testing and Clinical Outcomes in ED Chest Pain patients", *JAMA Intern Med*, 177(8), August 2017, https://jamanetwork.com/journals/jamainternalmedicine/fullarticle/2633257

[13] KS Dhillon, "Spinal Fusion for Chronic Low Back Pain: a "Magic Bullet' or Wishful Thinking?" *Malays Orthop.* J 2016 Mar; 10:(1):61-68 https://www.ncbi.nlm.nih.gov/pmc/articles/PMC5333707/

[14] Lila MacLellan, "The $100 billion per year back pain industry is mostly a hoax" *Quartz*, June 26, 2017, https://qz.com/1010259/the-100-billion-per-year-back-pain-industry-is-mostly-a-hoax/

20 percent.[15] That means more treatment and, in up to 25 percent of cases, a second operation.[16] A study published in the *Journal of the American Medical Association (JAMA)* found that hospitals take in an average of more than $30,000 in extra money per patient if there are post-surgical complications, and those complications can quadruple a person's length of hospital stay.[17]

A friend of mine from Washington, D.C., recently called with a story that puts all this into bold relief. A decade ago, her husband – I'll call him S.B. learned he had a common heart condition called atrial fibrillation, coupled with a poorly performing heart valve. His top-notch personal cardiologist evaluated him carefully and recommended he proceed slowly. But a second team at a renowned hospital thought he should undergo a more complicated open-heart surgery to repair the valve and perform an ablation "Maze" procedure to treat his atrial fibrillation. (In ablation, or Maze, tissue is scarred in order to disrupt faulty electrical signals that can cause an arrhythmia.) While the procedure was involved, he was told to expect to be back at work within the week.

---

[15] Nassau R, "Complications in Spine Surgery" *J Neurosurg Spine 2010 Aug;13(2), 144-57. doi: 10.3171/2010.3.SPINE09369.*
[16] Leonello Tacconi, "Lumbar discectomy: has it got any ill-effects?",*J. Spine Surg*, 2018 Sep 4(3): 677–680.doi: 10.21037/jss.2018.07.05 https://www.ncbi.nlm.nih.gov/pmc/articles/PMC6261748/
[17] Denise Grady, MD, "Hospitals Profit from Surgical Errors, Study Finds," *NYT*, 4/16/13 https://www.nytimes.com/2013/04/17/health/hospitals-profit-from-surgical-errors-study-finds.html

Instead, an unexpected complication required the subsequent placement of a pacemaker, which S.B. will need for the rest of his life in order for his heart to beat properly. Over the succeeding twelve-year period, the pacemaker wires fractured twice, necessitating two further surgeries. After the last operation, S.B. experienced a different, but potentially lethal heart rhythm. He has been wearing a LifeVest external defibrillator for the past three months to keep him safe, while he awaits a fourth surgery. His medical bills have topped $225,000.

The kicker: It's possible none of this would have happened had S.B. simply been treated from the get-go with medication for his abnormal heart rhythm. In fact, the CABANA study, published in *JAMA* 2019, found that whether a patient took medicine or underwent an ablation procedure, the outcomes were the same with respect to death, disabling stroke, heart attack, and serious bleeding.[18] And, in a survey of more than 33,000 ablation procedures to treat atrial fibrillation, complications occurred in every eighth or ninth patient — a 11 percent to 13 percent rate.[19]

Were the complications S.B. experienced fully discussed? I know

---

[18] Douglas Packer, "The CABANA Randomized Trial", *JamaNetwork*, March 15, 2019. doi:10.1001/jama.2019.0693.
https://jamanetwork.com/jour-%20nals/jama/fullarticle/2728676
[19] Gerhard Steinbeck, "Incidence of complications related to catheter ablation in atrial fibrillation and atrial flutter," *European Heart Journal*, Volume 39, Issue 45, 01 December 2018 https://academic.oup.com/eurheartj/article/39/45/4020/5063863

he did not know a permanent pacemaker was a possible outcome. For that matter, why do some doctors recommend more aggressive courses of therapy than others? Were the second hospital's physicians practicing in a different culture than S.B.'s cardiologist? Did the institution stand to benefit financially? Or, was it some combination of factors?

Overaggressive, unnecessary treatment can lead to patient harm, re-operations, longer stays, more studies, more tests, more imaging at a high cost to the patient. Meanwhile, the money rolls in for three significant players: hospitals, Big Pharma and medical device manufacturers.

Often, when patients find themselves steered toward a particular line of treatment — a certain medication, say, or a procedure calling for a specific brand of device — their doctors make these recommendations based on studies from the medical literature that appear to support the plan. In truth, those studies may well have been bought and paid for by the product's manufacturer.

Our medical literature is often fraught with bias in favor of certain products, because the drug and medical device companies sponsor so much of the research, and because their methods often deliberately lack rigor. A large study that included 370 randomized drug trials from a preeminent research review organization, Cochrane, concluded that industry-sponsored research was three times more likely to recommend the sponsor's drug as the preferred treatment than studies funded by nonprofits. They concluded this may be due to researchers' "biased interpretation of trial results."[20]

Biased data often becomes scientific fact. Not until independent researchers later repeat these trials with better controlled and higher-powered studies do they find that the purported benefit is

---

[20] Als-Nielsen, "Association of funding and conclusions in randomized drug trials: a reflection of treatment effect or adverse events? *JAMA*. 2003 Aug 20;290(7):921-8 https://pubmed.ncbi.nlm.nih.gov/12928469/

lacking, and the prior study's conclusions are reversed. A 10-year survey of research articles published in the *New England Journal of Medicine* showed that 40 percent of established medical practices were later found to be untrue.[21] By the time the medical community realizes a drug doesn't work, Big Pharma has made its money and moved on to promoting the next drug.

Do you take a statin, like Lipitor or Crestor, despite being an otherwise healthy person? The statin industry, remarkably lucrative in the U.S. on the premise that they can help prevent a first heart attack (in addition to its uses for those who already have coronary heart disease), is an example of where the effectiveness of and need for a medicine have been subject to tests with wildly differing conclusions.[22]

One meta-analysis by Kausik Ray, MD, et al., involving 65,000 patients, concluded that statins do not offer mortality benefit to people without heart disease, who use it as a preventative medicine.[23]

---

[21] Vinay Prasad, "A Decade of Reversal: An Analysis of 146 Contradicted Medical Practices", August 2013 Volume 88, Issue 8, 790–798, DOI:
https://www.mayoclinicproceedings.org/article/S0025-6196(13)00405-9/fulltext
[22] Michael Nedelman, "Should you take statins? Guidelines offer different answers" *CNN.com* Jan. 1 2018 https://www.cnn.com/2017/04/18/health/statins-guidelines-conflict-study/index.html
[23] Kausik Ray, "Statins and All-Cause Mortality in High-Risk Primary Prevention", *Arch Intern Med.* 2010;170(12):1024-1031. doi:10.1001/archinternmed.2010.182. https://jamanetwork.com/journals/jamainternalmedicine/fullarticle/416105

The drugs have been credibly linked to an increased risk of diabetes,[24] memory loss,[25] and muscle weakness.[26] Yet they continue to be prescribed and taken by some 35 million Americans.

The pharmaceutical industry has two primary pathways to achieve these elevated sales figures: paying for and thus controlling the results of research, and mass-marketing to physicians via gifts, free drug samples, research grants, paid speaking engagements, and more.

And they're not subtle: One company, Medtronic, sponsored 13 different studies that supported the use of its bone-growth product Infuse to improve outcomes for various back surgeries. None of the 13 trials reported any complications.[27] But in an independent article published in the *Journal of Spine*, Dr. Eugene Carragee of Stanford University reported "frequent and occasionally

---

[24] Sattar, N, "Statins and risk of incident diabetes: a collaborative meta-analysis of randomised statin trials." *Lancet*. 2010 Feb 27;375(9716):735-42. doi: 10.1016/S0140-6736(09)61965-6. Epub 2010 Feb 16. https://pubmed.ncbi.nlm.nih.gov/20167359/
[25] Chan AK, Fornazaari L, Golas AC, et al."Lipophilic statin use associated with deficits in memory and cognition." Presented at: 2018 Alzheimer's Association International Conference. July 22-26, 2018; Chicago, IL. Poster P2-586. https://www.neurologyadvisor.com/conference-highlights/aaic-2018/some-statins-may-be-associated-with-cognition-memory-deficits/
[26] Sabine Latteau, "A Mechanism for Statin-Induced Susceptibility to Myopathy", *JACC: Basic to Translational Science*, 2019; 4 (4): 509 https://www.sciencedaily.com/releases/2019/08/190826191928.htm
[27] "Staff Report on Medtronic's Influence on Infuse Clinical Studies." Prepared by the staff of the Committee on Finance United States Senate. 112th Congress, October 2012 https://www.finance.senate.gov/imo/media/doc/Medtronic_Report1.pdf

catastrophic complications" associated with Infuse's use in spinal fusion surgeries.[28] In his published review of the original data, Carragee estimated adverse events to range from 10 percent to 50 percent.

Additionally, physicians often used InFuse off-label in neck fusion surgeries; here the FDA found that some patients were experiencing life-threatening neck swelling and breathing difficulties.[29] You wouldn't know it from Medtronic's studies; the company paid the authors of the studies $210 million for "consulting, royalty, and other miscellaneous arrangements" over a 14-year period and "was heavily involved in drafting, editing and shaping" the content written by its paid experts, according to a U.S. Senate Committee on Finance.[30]

Years later, data from an internal large-scale review of Infuse outcomes – which Medtronic conducted – resurfaced in 2013 after being misplaced for more than 5 years, according to the Star-Tribune newspaper in Minneapolis. At the FDA's request for a list of "unreported serious injury events," Medtronic submitted a

---

[28] Eugene Caragee, A Critical Review of Recombinant Human Bone Morphoge- netic protein-2 Trials in Spinal Surgery: Emerging Safety Concerns and Lessons Learned, *Spine J*, Jun 11, 2011 (6):471-91 https://pubmed.ncbi.nlm.nih.gov/21729796/
[29] Eugene Caragee, *Spine J*, June 11, 2011 https://pubmed.ncbi.nlm.nih.gov/21729796/
[30] "Staff Report on Medtronic's Influence on Infuse Clinical Studies." Prepared by the staff of the Committee on Finance United States Senate. 112th Congress, October 2012 https://www.finance.senate.gov/imo/media/doc/Medtronic_Report1.pdf

summary which included 1,923 individual complications among 1,039 surgeries. Two or more complications were found in half of the surgeries.[31]

"OUR COMPANY HAS A DRAFT COMPLETE, WE JUST NEED AN AUTHOR," the progress note to Parke-Davis read in all capital letters. In "The Truth About the Drug Companies," Dr. Marcia Angell describes via whistleblower testimony how the drug manufacturer Warner-Lambert allegedly conducted an extensive, illegal marketing campaign through its Parke-Davis subsidiary to promote its drug Neurontin.[32] Supported by thousands of pages of company documents, whistleblower David Franklin described how Parke-Davis hired outside companies to ghostwrite journal articles with little data, then paid academicians to "author" them. By heavily promoting Neurontin's benefit for multiple unapproved uses – by 2000, 78 percent of the drug's prescriptions written were for off-label use – the company expanded its market, and Neurontin sales skyrocketed.[33]

Pfizer, which had acquired Warner-Lambert in 2000, ultimately

---

[31] Joe Carlson and Jim Spencer, "Lost Medtronic data showed serious risks with Infuse surgical implant", Star Tribune, December 16, 2108
https://www.startribune.com/lost-medtronic-report-showed-serious-risks-with-infuse-surgical-implant/502798952/
[32] Dr Marcia Angell. The Truth About the Drug Companies. *Random House Books*, 2004
[33] Christian Krautkramer, "Neurontin and Off-Label Marketing," *AMA J. of Ethics*, Jun 2006. https://emcrit.org/pulmcrit/actt-remdesivir/

pled guilty to falsely misbranding Neurontin and settled criminal charges incurred by Medicaid fraud.[34] Noted U.S. Attorney Michael Sullivan, "This illegal and fraudulent promotion scheme corrupted the information process relied upon by doctors in their medical decision-making, thereby putting patients at risk."[35] Criminal and civil liabilities totaled $430 million; sales of the drug were $2.7 billion in 2003 alone.

We have to ask ourselves what is happening during this coronavirus pandemic, as multiple pharmaceutical companies have been conducting their own studies and publishing much of their own data — some without peer review — in respected medical journals. For example, we've heard a lot about the drug Remdesevir in the media as a potential treatment option for COVID-19 patients. Josh Farkas, M.D., editor of *PulmCrit.org* points out that in the first randomized control trial of Remdesivir use, published in the *New England Journal of Medicine*, the study was "designed, conducted, analyzed, and written by Gilead Sciences" the maker of the drug.[36] He also describes several other problems, including the authors changing the primary endpoint of

---

[34] Christian Krautkramer, "Neurontin and Off-Label Marketing," *AMA J. of Ethics*, June 2006. https://emcrit.org/pulmcrit/actt-remdesivir/
[35] Dept. of Justice: Warner-Lambert to pay $430 million to resolve criminal & civil health care liability relating to off-label promotion, May 13, 2004. https://www.justice.gov/archive/opa/pr/2004/May/04_civ_322.htm
[36] Josh Farkas, "Preliminary report on NIAID trial of Remdesivir (ACTT-1)", *Pulmcrit.org*. May 23, 2020. https://emcrit.org/pulmcrit/actt-remdesivir/

the study, the study lacking several secondary endpoints, and it missing a very basic component: a placebo group for comparison. Does Gilead fear that taking Remdesivir might not be better than taking nothing at all?

Interestingly, World Health Organization experts reported interim results seven months later in the *New England Journal of Medicine* of a very large multinational trial performed at 45 hospitals in 30 countries comprising thousands of patients.[37] The upshot: They found no mortality benefit in the group given Remdesivir versus the control group. In fact, the death rates were nearly identical. Neither did the drug shorten patients' hospital stay or affect their chances of ending up on a breathing machine. While a previous trial had shown that Remdesivir improved patients' recovery time in the hospital, this much larger trial showed little effect.[38] [39]

What are the typical charges for Remdesivir for insured patients? Try $3,120 for a patient receiving a shorter, typical course of the

---

[37] WHO Solidarity Rial Consortium, "Repurposed Antiviral Drugs for Covid-19 00 Interim WHO Solidarity Trial Results, *N Engl J Med*, December 2, 2020. https://www.nejm.org/doi/full/10.1056/NEJMoa2023184

[38] Anthony Bavry, Adaptive COVID-19 Treatment Trial – ACTT-1", American College of Cardiology https://www.acc.org/latest-in-cardiology/clinical-trials/2020/10/12/23/32/actt-1

[39] WHO Solidarity Rial Consortium, "Repurposed Antiviral Drugs for Covid-19 00 Interim WHO Solidarity Trial Results, N Engl J Med, December 2, 2020. https://www.nejm.org/doi/full/10.1056/NEJMoa2023184

medication; and $5,270 for one receiving a longer course.[40] These numbers might help explain why, according to RBC Capital Markets analyst Brian Abrahams, Remdesivir sales could reach $2.3 billion this year, with $1.3 billion profit.[41]

The implications of all this are obvious: When you control the research, you control the information, the conclusions, the market and the money.

A *New England Journal of Medicine* article found that negative studies on the effects of antidepressants were routinely not published.[42] The result? The available research (that is, the things that *were* published) suggested that 94 percent of the antidepressant trials were positive. In fact, once all the FDA registered studies were factored (including unpublished trials), the authors found that only 51 percent of the trials were positive. Would you take an antidepressant knowing that it was a coin-flip as to whether it would actually help, but a 100 percent guarantee that any side effects would hurt you?

---

[40] Joseph Walker, "Covid-19 Drug Remdesivir to Cost $3,120 for Typical Patient," *WSJ*, June 29, 2020 https://www.wsj.com/articles/covid-19-drug-remdesivir-to-cost-3-120-for-typical-patient-11593428402

[41] Joseph Walker, "Covid-19 Drug Remdesivir to Cost $3,120 for Typical Patient," *WSJ*, June 29, 2020 https://www.wsj.com/articles/covid-19-drug-remdesivir-to-cost-3-120-for-typical-patient-11593428402

[42] Erick Turner, "Selective Publication of Antidepressant Trials and Its Influence on Apparent Efficacy", *N Engl J Med 2008*; 358:252-260 DOI: 10.1056/NEJMsa065779. https://www.nejm.org/doi/full/10.1056/NEJMsa065779#t=abstract

Well-meaning physicians, searching for the right answers for their patients, can make inappropriate decisions based on such manipulated research. We often are guided by what we know or read. But the concept of evidence-based medicine, for so long a sort of hallmark of trustworthiness, appears to have been disturbingly corrupted by drug and device manufacturers whose deep pockets can change the results and the reporting.[43]

Sometimes they influence the doctors themselves. The federally administered website Open Payments calculates that pharmaceutical and medical device company payments to doctors and teaching hospitals exceeded $9 billion in 2018 alone.[44] More than two billion dollars of that money went to speaking and consulting fees, meals, travel and gifts. Even a medium-size drug company like Forest Labs spent $32 million for paid speeches in 2013.[45] While approximately half of the doctors accepted money from industry in 2015,[46] Open Payments Data reveals that 627,000 doctors — an increase to 68% — received some form of

---

[43] Jason Fung, "The Corruption of Evidence Based Medicine — Killing for Profit", *Medium.com*, April 10, 2018 https://drjasonfung.medium.com/the-corruption-of-evidence-based-medicine-killing-for-profit-41f2812b8704
[44] OpenPaymentsData, Published on January 17, 2020, https://openpaymentsdata.cms.gov/summary
[45] Charles Ornstein, "How Much Are Drug Companies Paying Your Doctor?" *Sci. American*, Sept 30, 2014. https://www.scientificamerican.com/article/how-much-are-drug-companies-paying-your-doctor/
[46] Dennis Thompson, "Survey reveals how many doctors receive money, gifts from drugmakers" *CBSNews*, May 3, 2017

industry payment in 2018.[47]

Though Big Pharma's marketing tentacles extend into every field of medicine, oncology is particularly appealing prey, with medications that can run from $150,000 to $250,000 per patient, per year.[48] The drugmaker Merck, for example, recently announced it is spinning off $6.5 billion in assets to focus on higher-margin segments — that is, faster sales-growth areas — like cancer drugs.[49] Partly because of that focus and partly due to scientific and regulatory issues, our pipeline of (lower profit) antibiotics for novel agents has all but dried up: Few new classes of antibiotics have been developed since 1984; and no new class has been developed for the deadly multidrug resistant gram negative superbugs since 1962![50] [51]

Oncologists have a unique arrangement that allows them to purchase intravenous chemotherapy and immunotherapy drugs

---

[47] Mike Tigas, "Dollars for Docs: How Industry Dollars Reached Your Doctors" *ProPublica*, Oct 17, 2019. https://projects.propublica.org/docdollars/
[48] Deana Beasley, "The cost of cancer: new drugs show success at a steep price", *Reuters, Health News*, April, 3, 2017. https://www.reuters.com/article/us-usa-healthcare-cancer-costs/the-cost-of-cancer-new-drugs-show-success-at-a-steep-price-idUSKBN1750FU
[49] Jared Hopkins, "Merck to Spin Off Slow-Growth Products Into New Company", The *Wall Street Journal*, February 5, 2020. https://www.wsj.com/articles/merck-to-spin-off-slow-growth-products-into-new-company-11580903102
[50] "Antibacterial agents in clinical Development," *World Health Organization* ,2019. https://apps.who.int/iris/bitstream/handle/10665/330420/9789240000193-eng.pdf
[51] Tim Links, "Why is it so difficult to discover new antibiotics?" *BBC News*, Oct. 27, 2017. https://www.bbc.com/news/health-41693229

wholesale from pharmacies, mark up the prices, and then bill insurance companies or patients at a profit. The more expensive the drug, the greater the profit. Researchers at Harvard found that when Medicare reimbursements for a lung cancer drug called paclitaxel dropped markedly, but reimbursement of a similar drug remained the same, oncologists switched to prescribing the more expensive drug.[52] Moreover, the pharmaceutical industry can influence which drug an oncologist chooses by discounting its wholesale cost to improve the physician's margin.

In a similar scheme, the industry giant TAP Pharmaceuticals settled a healthcare fraud case for $875 million: It allegedly charged Medicare and other insurers approximately $500 per dose for a prostate cancer drug called Lupron, but allowed physicians to buy it for $350 to $400 and pocket the difference.[53] Moving those margins meant increasing sales of the drug and mass profits for the company.

Smaller money matters, too. A 2018 *JAMA* study showed that oncologists who received any industry payment over $10 were twice as likely to prescribe that drug company's medicine for

---

[52] Peter Ubel, MD, "Do oncologists have an incentive to prescribe expensive treatments?" *KevinMD.com*, July 4, 2012.
https://www.kevinmd.com/blog/2012/07/oncologists-incentive-prescribe-expensive-treatments.html
[53] "TAP Pharmaceuticals Agrees to Pay Record $875M Fine in Medicare, Medicaid Fraud Case" *KHN.org*, June 11, 2009 https://khn.org/morning-breakout/dr00007291/

metastatic kidney cancer patients, and 29 percent more likely to prescribe its medicine for chronic myeloid leukemia patients.[54] Spreading money works. Across all specialties, a *ProPublica* 2019 analysis of fifty popular medications found that doctors who received payments linked to drugs from Big Pharma, wrote 58% more prescriptions of that drug, on average, than physicians without these ties.[55]

Oncologists often run clinical trials to evaluate the efficacy of different drug regimens on cancer patients — but this, too, can be an area of conflict, because the doctors may get paid "finder's fees" and bonus payments for patient recruitment, totaling tens of thousands of dollars, from the drug manufacturers themselves.[56]

Considering how desperate many end-stage cancer patients often feel, and how easily they might be talked into a trial without knowing all the possible side effects, this scenario creates a

---

[54] Mia de Graaf, "Cancer doctors are twice as likely to pick one drug over another if they got kickbacks from the manufacturer, study reveals" *Daily Mail*, April 9, 2018 https://www.dailymail.co.uk/health/article-5595025/Cancer-doctors-TWICE-likely-pick-one-drug-got-kickbacks.html

[55] Hannah Fresques, "Doctors Prescribe More of a Drug If They Receive Money from a Pharma Company Tied to It", *ProPublica*, Dec 20, 2019.
https://www.propublica.org/article/doctors-prescribe-more-of-a-drug-if-they-receive-money-from-a-pharma-company-tied-to-it

[56] U Penn: "Institutional Review Board Payment for Referral/Recruitment of Subjects in Human Research" https://irb.upenn.edu/sites/default/files/payment-for-recruitment-of-subjects-guidance.pdf

serious ethical conundrum. And the wheels come off entirely when patients are often being roped into experimental trials with quite unproven benefits: Vinay Prasad, Assistant Professor at the University of California San Francisco, reported in 2017 that two-thirds of cancer medicines that are prescribed and fully FDA-approved over the past two years do not increase survival at all.[57] A recently published study, meanwhile, found that of 92 cancer drugs approved by the FDA from 2000 to 2016, the median overall survival for patients increased by only 2.4 months.[58] Additionally, only about half of the studies relied on evidence from randomized trials; approved data showed that both doctors and patients typically had access to limited information regarding the possible benefits of these new cancer therapies when the drugs came on the market.

And like lawyers picking a jury, pharmaceutical companies often use carefully defined exclusion criteria to "cherry pick" participants for these trials. The study participants chosen are generally younger and healthier, with fewer comorbidities (pre-existing conditions) than people who use these drugs in the real

---

[57] Liz Szabo, "Amid flurry of new cancer drugs, how many offer real benefits?" *CNN.com*, Feb. 9, 2017,
https://www.cnn.com/2017/02/09/health/hope-vs-hype-cancer-drugs-partner/index.html
[58] Aviv Ladanie, Andreas Schmitt, Benjamin Speich, et al. "Clinical Trial Evidence Supporting US Food and Drug Administration Approval of Novel Cancer Therapies Between 2000 and 2016," *JAMA Network*, November 10, 2020
https://jamanetwork.com/journals/jamanetworkopen/fullarticle/2772736

world.[59] In a recent study in *JAMA Oncology* looking at the ages of more than 260,000 participants in 302 trials for various types of cancers, researchers found the participants were much younger than that of the real-world population with disease.[60] Age disparity was also associated with industry-funded research. Consequently, results from these carefully designed trials often yield more favorable results — for Big Pharma, that is.[61]

It bears repeating that under the best conditions with the drug companies throwing money into these trials, the results are still generally mediocre. Some 92 new cancer drugs that were approved over a 17-year period, for example, improved mortality for cancer patients across the board by only about two and a half months. And those results, remember, came through carefully designed research trials. Imagine the poor survival odds of patients seen in our hospital clinics every day who may be older, sicker or have pre-existing co-morbidities, or of patients who

---

[59] Pratibha Gopalakrishna "New research shows older adults are still often excluded from clinical trials," *STAT*, September 30, 2020
https://www.statnews.com/2020/09/30/age-disparities-clinical-trials-covid19/

[60] Ethan Ludmir, MD, Walker Mainwaring, Timothy Lin, et al. "Factors Associated with Age Disparities Among Cancer Clinical Trial Particpants, *JAMA Oncology*, June 3, 2019,
https://jamanetwork.com/journals/jamaoncology/fullarticle/10.1001/jamaoncol.2019.2055

[61] Ben Goldacre, "Trial sans Error: How Pharma-Funded Research Cherry-Picks Positive Results," *Scientific American*, February 13, 2013
https://www.scientificamerican.com/article/trial-sans-error-how-pharma-funded-research-cherry-picks-positive-results/

enroll in untested clinical trials.[62]

On almost every page of its 2019 guidelines to physicians, the National Comprehensive Cancer Network (NCCN) has displayed in a separately boxed area, in bold, the following statement: "NCCN believes that the best management of any cancer patient is in a clinical trial. Participation in clinical trials is especially encouraged." Why? Is it really in the best interest of every patient — or even most patients?

Big Pharma and hospitals do need patients enrolled in the more than 300,000 clinical trials now being conducted globally.[63] But, there's a catch: many of these trials are not investigating novel treatments that patients might hope will save their lives, but rather "me-too" drugs which are copycats of existing medications. It is much cheaper for pharmaceutical manufacturers to bring me-too drugs to market, apply for new patents, heavily market the drugs as the "latest and greatest", and let the money roll in.[64] Novel drug development is much costlier and riskier — and therefore far less

---

[62] Szabo, "Amid flurry of new cancer drugs, how many offer real benefits?" *CNN.com*, Feb. 9, 2017 https://www.cnn.com/2017/02/09/health/hope-vs-hype-cancer-drugs-partner/index.html
[63] Matej Mikulic, "Total Number of registered studies worldwide" Statista, October 10, 2019 https://www.statista.com/statistics/732997/number-of-registered-clinical-studies-worldwide/
[64] Rosanne Spector, "Sometimes they're just the same old, same old", *Stanford Medicine Magazine*, Summer 2005,
http://sm.stanford.edu/archive/stanmed/2005summer/drugs-metoo.html

common.

In her book, Dr. Marcia Angell, a former editor-in-chief of the *NEJM*, noted that from 1998 to 2002, 77% of the 415 FDA-approved new medications were copycats. If a similar percentage holds true today, a patient subjected to all the risks and harms of a clinical trial has a three in four chance of receiving a drug that is virtually identical to ones already on the market.[65] Patients do not know this. Many doctors do not know this. It is important that investigators and institutions mitigate conflicts of interest when enrolling patients in clinical trials by being completely forthright with any payments they may be receiving, and by offering full disclosure with respect to trial options, the risks and benefits, and the likelihoods of failure.[66]

Understand: Most physicians are good doctors, honest, hard-working, who are trying to practice medicine within strict ethical boundaries. But it's critically important to remember that the pharmaceutical, biotech, and medical device industries, while advancing many great drugs and products, are also very good salespeople.

---

[65] Marcia Angell, MD, The Truth About the Drug Companies. *Random House Books*, Aug 9, 2005.
[66] Miney Paquette, "Ethical issues in competing clinical trials" *Contemp Clin Trials Commun*. 2019 Jun; 14: 100352.
https://www.ncbi.nlm.nih.gov/pmc/articles/PMC6461579/

From the time a doctor is a medical student, and continuing throughout his or her residency and career, industry marketers cater lunches, bring gifts, offer free gatherings at expensive restaurants under the guise of "medical training," and fund national conferences. These meetings can be gatherings of 5,000 to 10,000 physicians from all over the world. They provide an excellent opportunity for the industry to showcase its drugs, or even pay prominent leaders in the field to give canned marketing lectures, which, subtly or more blatantly, promote that company's drug or device.

As a physician gains seniority, the industry has more financially rewarding means of influence. A doctor may not only be hired for speaking engagements where travel, hotel expenses, and a speaking fee in the $2,000 to $10,000 range are all paid, but he or she may also be paid six figures to sit on a pharmaceutical or device company's advisory board. A physician may even be given stock options or receive patent royalties from an invention.

Does the industry's involvement work? Far too often, it appears to work like a charm. Consider the clot-busting drug tissue plasminogen activator (tPA), which was developed as a medication for stroke victims. Despite strong controversy among physicians about the drug's efficacy (in only two of twelve studies did it show a benefit), the drug was assigned a Class I "definitely recommend" status by the American Heart Association.[67] Turns out, six of the nine stroke experts who wrote the new guidelines had financial ties to tPA's manufacturer, Genentech, which also had contributed $11 million to the AHA. Did that help persuade the drug's use? I can't imagine it hurt.

There are darker stories too — stories of outright mail and wire fraud, bribery, and racketeering. Alec Burlakoff, a former senior executive at Insys Therapeutics,[68] told *60 Minutes* in June that the company paid bribes to physicians — up to $125,000 a year, he said — so that the doctors would prescribe more of the Insys opioid painkiller drug Subsys.[69]

The payments were disguised as speaker fees. Company sales representatives instructed the physicians, "The more prescriptions you write, the more you're going to earn. And, the more you increase the strength (of the drug), the more you're going to earn."[70]

---

[67] David Newman, "Thrombolytics for Acute Ischemic Stroke," *Thennt.com*, March 25, 2013, https://www.thennt.com/nnt/thrombolytics-for-stroke/

[68] US Dept of Justice: "Opioid Manufacturer Insys Therapeutics Agrees to Enter $225 Million Global Resolution of Criminal and Civil Investigations." June 5, 2019. https://www.justice.gov/opa/pr/opioid-manufacturer-insys-therapeutics-agrees-enter-225-million-global-resolution-criminal

[69] Mabel Kabani, "Alec Burlakoff: The rise and fall of a pharmaceutical opioid sales executive." *60 Minutes*, June 21, 2020. https://www.cbsnews.com/news/alec-burlakoff-rise-and-fall-of-a-pharmaceutical-opioid-sales-executive-60-minutes-2020-06-21/

[70] Mabel Kabani, "Alec Burlakoff" *60 Minutes*, June 21, 2020

The speaker-fee gambit is not unusual — in fact, it's a common and very lucrative one. According to a November 2020 Officer of Inspector General (OIG) special fraud alert, pharmaceutical and medical device companies paid nearly $2 billion for healthcare speaker-related services over the last three years.[71] The OIG and Department of Justice (DOJ) have "investigated and resolved numerous fraud cases involving allegations that remuneration offered and paid in connection with speaker programs violated the anti-kickback statute." The alert cautioned that speaker programs may be subject to increased scrutiny going forward and warned physicians that an improper consulting arrangement with a drug or device company could "violate fraud and abuse laws."[72]

US Attorney Andrew E. Lelling accused Insys of engaging in "prolonged, illegal conduct that prioritized its profits over the health of thousands of patients." The landmark criminal case, Lelling said, meant the company was finally being held accountable for its role in fueling the opioid epidemic.[73]

---

[71] Office of Inspector General, "Special Fraud Alert: Speaker Programs", *Dept. Of Health and Human Services*, November 16, 2020. https://oig.hhs.gov/fraud/docs/alertsandbulletins/2020/SpecialFraudAlertSpeakerPrograms.pdf

[72] Office of Inspector General, "Special Fraud Alert: Speaker Programs," *Dept. Of Health and Human Services*, November 16, 2020 https://oig.hhs.gov/fraud/docs/alertsandbulletins/2020/SpecialFraudAlertSpeakerPrograms.pdf

[73] US Dept of Justice, June 5, 2019. https://www.justice.gov/opa/pr/opioid-manu-%20facturer-insys-therapeutics-agrees-enter-225-million-global-resolution-criminal

Likewise, Novartis Pharmaceutical Corp. recently settled for $678 million a fraud lawsuit in which prosecutors alleged that over a nine-year-period, the company paid kickbacks to physicians so that they would overprescribe Novartis' drugs. The kickbacks came in the form of "cash, meals, alcohol, hotels, travel, entertainment, and honoraria payments." Some Novartis sales representatives targeted high-prescribing doctors to become speakers, paying them tens or hundreds of thousands of dollars in honoraria, with the understanding that they would write more prescriptions. According to the U.S. District Court documents, one physician received a total of $320,000, and wrote more than 8,000 prescriptions for the company's drugs.

For Novartis, it wasn't the first time. The firm settled a similar claim in 2010, after U.S. attorneys alleged that over a seven-year period, the company had provided "illegal remuneration to doctors through mechanisms such as speaker programs, advisory boards, and gifts," violating the Anti-Kickback Statue. But perhaps paying millions in fines is simply a line-item in the cost of doing business: Last year, the company generated $47.7 billion in revenue.

Nearly 25 years since the introduction of Oxycontin, Purdue Pharma pled guilty to three federal felonies related to the marketing and distribution of its addictive prescription painkiller, agreeing to pay an $8.34 billion settlement.[74] The criminal charges included conspiring to defraud U.S. officials and paying illegal kickbacks to physicians through speakers' fees that induced them to write more opioid prescriptions.

When OxyContin came on the market in the mid-1990's, Purdue aggressively promoted the drug as one with a low potential for addiction, "less than one percent."[75] This was untrue, which the company knew and later admitted in a 2007 criminal lawsuit that resulted in it paying a $635 million fine.[76] Physicians, however, were unaware for many years and continued to prescribe, and overprescribe it, with many patients becoming addicted.

As part of a multifaceted, aggressive marketing campaign, Purdue awarded large bonuses to sales representatives who sold more Oxycontin in their respective regions. They often achieved this by specifically targeting the highest prescribing physicians in the country.[77] Further, the company aggressively promoted the use of their drug for chronic non-cancer related pain — a much larger

---

[74] Sara Randazzo, Purdue Pharma Pleads Guilty to Felonies Over its OxyContin Sales," *WSJ*, November, 25, 2020 https://www.wsj.com/articles/purdue-pharma-pleads-guilty-to-felonies-over-oxycontin-sales-11606243071
[75] Art Van Zee, MD "The Promotion and Marketing of OxyContin: Commercial Triumph, Public Health Tragedy. *Am J Public Health* ,February 2009, https://www.nature.com/articles/d41586-019-02686-2
[76] Art Van Zee, MD *Am J Public Health,* February 2009.
[77] Art Van Zee, MD *Am J Public Health*, February 2009

market, but one for which efficacy and use is much less clear.[78] This resulted in a nearly tenfold increase in OxyContin prescriptions for this type of pain over a 5-year period.[79] Said Drug Enforcement Administration assistant Tim McDermott, "The devastating ripple effect of Purdue's actions left lives lost and others addicted."[80]

Yet, back in an email in February 2001, as questions were starting to be raised about OxyContin, Dr. Richard Sackler, former president and chairman of Purdue Pharma, directed blame to those who had become addicted: "We have to hammer on the abusers in every way possible. They are the culprits and the problem. They are reckless criminals."[81] It took more than two decades for Purdue Pharma to finally acknowledge its role in fueling the opioid epidemic that has killed now almost 450,000 people from 1999-2018.[82]

Since doctors not only write prescriptions, but also provide patient

---

[78] Art Van Zee, MD *Am J Public Health* February 2009
[79] Art Van Zee, MD *Am J Public Health*, February 2009
[80] John Fauber, "Purdue Pharma, Whose OxyContin helped fuel the opioid epidemic," agrees to pay $8 billion," *Milwaukee Journal Sentinel*, October 21, 2020
https://www.jsonline.com/story/news/2020/10/21/opioid-epidemic-oxycontin-maker-purdue-pharma-settles-lawsuit/3715885001/
[81] Andrew Joseph, "'A Blizzard of prescriptions': Documents reveal new details about Purdue's marketing of OxyContin." *Stat News*, January 15, 2019
https://www.statnews.com/2019/01/15/massachusetts-purdue-lawsuit-new-details/
[82] "Understanding the Epidemic," *Center for Disease Control*,
https://www.cdc.gov/drugoverdose/epidemic/index.html

referrals, drug and device companies may likewise target them in other kickback schemes. DaVita Healthcare Partners, which operates 2625 dialysis centers, was accused of entering into precisely such ventures with kidney doctors at 26 dialysis clinics over a nine-year period. Said US Attorney John Walsh, "This case involved a sophisticated scheme to compensate doctors for referring patients to DaVita's dialysis centers."[83] Ultimately, DaVita paid $389 million in 2014 to settle a criminal and civil anti-kickback investigation, without admitting guilt.

Two companies, DaVita and Germany-headquartered Fresenius, own some 70 percent of the dialysis clinics in the U.S, each reporting an annual net income of approximately $1 billion.[84] DaVita's share of joint venture clinics has increased from 259 in 2008 to 671 in 2018.[85]

Jeffrey Berns, M.D., a nephrologist, has written extensively about the lack of transparency regarding such joint-venture

---

[83] Christopher Osher, "Devita to Pay 389 million to settle anti-kickback investigation." *Denver Post*, Oct 22, 2014 https://www.denverpost.com/2014/10/22/davita-to-pay-389-million-to-settle-anti-kickback-investigations/
[84] Jeffrey Berns, Aaron Glickman, and Matthew McCoy, "Dialysis-Facility Joint-Venture Ownership – Hidden Conflicts of Interest, " *NEJM*, October 4, 2018 https://www.nejm.org/doi/full/10.1056/NEJMp1805097
[85] Carrie Arnold, Larry Price, "Should your Kidney Doctor Have a Financial Stake in Dialysis?, *Scientific American*, December 15, 2020 https://www.scientificamerican.com/article/should-your-kidney-doctor-have-a-financial-stake-in-dialysis/

arrangements.[86] Shouldn't patients know whether their kidney doctor has a financial stake in a dialysis center when the physician is recommending that they start dialysis (as opposed to some other treatment that might work) and then referring them to that doctor's own dialysis treatment center, where the physician stands to profit?

"No one outside the few big chains that own most dialysis clinics has any idea how many are operated as joint ventures," said Berns, "and how that arrangement can influence medical decision-making." In a Scientific American article, he suggested that the partnership leaves many kidney doctors with a financial incentive to direct patients to dialysis centers, even when other options like diet, lifestyle changes or medications might have been satisfactory.[87]

A Marketdata report from July 2019 revealed that more than 7,500 dialysis clinics reported an average $3 million in annual receipts per clinic, an approximate net profit margin of 18 percent.[88] Said a colleague of Bern's at Penn, Matthew McCoy, PhD, "It's a classic case of conflict of interest. If you own a share in the

---

[86] Berns, NEJM 2018 https://www.nejm.org/doi/full/10.1056/NEJMp1805097
[87] Carrie Arnold, *Scientific American*, December 15, 2020
[88] John LaRosa, "US Kidney Dialysis Clinics Form a Profitable $24 Billion Industry," *Blog.MarketResearch.com* July 29, 2019 https://blog.marketresearch.com/u.s.-kidney-dialysis-clinics-form-a-profitable-24-billion-industry

facility, there's financial incentives to get patients there and keep them there."[89] And no law exists stating that physicians need to disclose their financial conflict to patients. Transparency is needed so patients can make fully informed medical decisions regarding their treatment options. [90]

The dialysis clinic situation is an example of something happening fully within the bounds of what is legally acceptable, though perhaps morally questionable, and we need to separate it from DaVita's referral-kickback scheme or Purdue Pharma's outrageous, felonious behavior that induced physicians to write more and more needless opioid prescriptions. Scams like these couldn't have happened without some bad actors on the physician side, but these take in a tiny percentage of doctors. The real danger to you as a patient lies in the ability of Big Pharma and the device manufacturers to influence not only prescribing practices, but also research and decision-making. Pharmaceutical companies spend more marketing to doctors than they do on the research and development of all new drugs. That may ultimately mean big profit, but it's also bad medicine.

---

[89] Carrie Arnold, *Scientific American*, December 15, 2020
[90] Jeffrey Berns, *NEJM*, October 4, 2018.

Speaking of bad medicine and profit, why do we spend so much on healthcare in the U.S. and why don't we have better outcomes to show for all that spending? We burn more money on healthcare than any other country, whether measured as a percentage of GDP[91] or per capita.[92] Our system leaves far too many patients saddled with huge medical expenses — and that's to say nothing of the millions among us who cannot afford coverage at all.[93] In fact, according to the 2018 National Financial Capability Study, 23% of Americans have unpaid, past-due medical bills and nearly 3 in 10 Americans have avoided seeking medical care due to cost concerns.[94] COVID-19's ravages have provided us an opportune moment to reflect on our broken system and decide how we want it to work for us.

First, let's talk about how we got here, because a significant part of the problem is that our healthcare system was never really

---

[91] Roosa Tikkanen & Melinda Abrams, "U.S. Health Care from a Global Perspective, 2019: Higher Spending, Worse Outcomes?" *The Commonwealth Fund*, January 30, 2020, https://www.commonwealthfund.org/publications/issue-briefs/2020/jan/us-health-care-global-perspective-2019

[92] "U.S Health Care Spending Highest Among Developed Countries" *Johns Hopkins Bloomberg School of Public Health*, January 7, 2019, https://www.jhsph.edu/news/news-releases/2019/us-health-care-spending-highest-among-developed-countries.html

[93] Jennifer Tolbert, Kendal Orgera & Anthony Damico, "Key Facts about the uninsured Population", *KFF.org*, November 6, 2020. https://www.kff.org/uninsured/issue-brief/key-facts-about-the-uninsured-population/

[94] Judy Lin, Christopher Bumcrot, Tippy Ulicny et al. "The State of U.S. Financial Capability: The 2018 National Financial Capability Study," *FINRA Investor Education Foundation* https://www.usfinancialcapability.org/downloads/NFCS_2018_Report_Natl_Findings.pdf

master-planned. During World War II, with the government restricting wage increases in order to fight inflation, businesses began creating employer-sponsored health insurance in order to attract new employees.[95] That practice continued through the decades, and our healthcare system evolved into what Brad Spellberg, chief medical officer at LAC + USC Medical Center, describes in his book *Broken, Bankrupt, and Dying* as a "hodgepodge" of uncoordinated care involving insurance companies, healthcare providers, and government programs.[96]

This makeshift system has cost us dearly.[97] Our healthcare expenditure in 2018 was $3.7 trillion, or 16.9% of GDP — nearly twice as expensive as that of the average Organization for Economic and Cooperation and Development (OECD) peer high-income countries.[98]

In a famous paper, Uwe Reinhardt, a Princeton economist who spent decades studying health reform, identified the reason for this

---

[95] Jeff Griffin, "The history of Medicine and Organized Healthcare in America," *JP Griffin Group*, March 27, 2020, https://www.griffinbenefits.com/blog/history-of-healthcare
[96] Brad Spellberg. Broken, Bankrupt, and Dying. Lioncrest Publishing 2020.
[97] William Shrank, Teresa Rogstad, Natasha Parekh, "Waste in the US Health Care System Estimated Costs and Potential for Savings," *JAMA Network*, October 7, 2019, https://jamanetwork.com/journals/jama/article-abstract/2752664
[98] Roosa Tikkanen & Melinda Abrams, "U.S. Health Care from a Global Perspective, 2019: Higher Spending, Worse Outcomes?" *The Commonwealth Fund*, January 30, 2020

excessive spending: "It's the prices, stupid."[99] Sixteen years later, a 2019 study by Johns Hopkins researchers came to a similar conclusion.[100] Higher pharmaceutical prices, hospital medical charges, physicians' and nurses' salaries, and administrative costs explained America's wild overspending on healthcare. That cost is expected to rise to $6 trillion by 2027.[101]

In the United States, we spend more per capita than any other country on prescriptions drugs — an average of about two times that of other peer nations.[102] According to OECD data, Americans spend about $1,200 per person on prescriptions drugs per year.[103] This may help explain why more than one in five American adults, or 58 million people, report that at some point over the last 12 months they could not pay for needed medications.[104]

---

[99] Gerard Anderson, Uwe Reinhardt, Peter S. Hussey and Varduhi Petrosyan, "It's the prices, Stupid: Why the US is so Different from other Countries," *HealthAffairs*, May/June 2003. https://www.healthaffairs.org/doi/full/10.1377/hlthaff.22.3.89
[100] "U.S Health Care Spending Highest Among Developed Countries" *Johns Hopkins Bloomberg School of Public Health*, January 7, 2019
https://www.jhsph.edu/news/news-releases/2019/us-health-care-spending-highest-among-developed-countries.html
[101] "Healthcare costs for Americans Projected to Grow at an Alarmingly High Rate," *Peter G. Peterson Foundation*, May 1, 2019
https://www.pgpf.org/blog/2019/05/healthcare-costs-for-americans-projected-to-grow-at-an-alarmingly-high-rate
[102] Yoni Bloomberg, "Here's why many prescription drugs in the US cost so much," CNBC, January 14, 2019
[103] "Pharmaceutical Spending", *OECD data*, 2019
https://data.oecd.org/healthres/pharmaceutical-spending.htm
[104] Chuck Grassley, "58 Million American Adults Can't Afford Prescription Drugs", *Grassley.senate.gov*, Nov 12, 2019 https://www.grassley.senate.gov/news/news-releases/icymi-58-million-american-adults-can-t-afford-prescription-drugs

And when considering price variation among countries, it's staggering how much more Americans are likely to pay. Humira, used to treat various inflammatory conditions costs $552 in South Africa, $822 in Switzerland, $1,362 in the U.K., but $2,669 in the U.S. — for the exact same drug.[105] A 30-day supply of a multiple sclerosis medication, Tecfidera, retails for approximately $5,089 in the U.S., compared to $663 in Great Britain.[106]

These aren't just aberrations — medicines and medical procedures in the U.S. routinely cost much more. According to an International Federation of Health Plan report and as reported by Vox: a hepatitis C medicine, Harvoni, costs $10,000 more in the US than in other countries; a cancer drug, Avastin, costs nine times more than it does in the U.K.; an MRI costs twice as much as it does in Switzerland and five times as much in Australia; a day in a hospital costs $5,220 in the U.S., but only $424 in Spain. Surgery to remove an appendix costs $12,000 more here than in Australia; a normal delivery of a baby costs over $10,000 here but just over $5,000 in Australia and about $2,000 in Spain; a C-section (cesarean delivery) is approximately $16,000, which is more than double the cost of the surgery in Australia and five

---

[105] Edwin Lopez, "Report: US drug prices often higher than in other developed countries", *BioPharmadive,* July 20, 2016
https://www.biopharmadive.com/news/report-us-drug-prices-often-higher-than-in-other-developed-countries/422959/
[106] Edwin Lopez, https://www.biopharmadive.com/news/report-us-drug-prices-often-higher-than-in-other-developed-countries/422959/

times the charges in Spain. Cardiac bypass surgery costs $78,318 here compared to $24,059 in the UK; and the same is true for knee replacements: $28,184 here versus $18,451 in the UK and only $6,687 in Spain.[107] While there are a few exceptions, we overspend for healthcare in the U.S.

Lack of price control strategies and cost ceilings may be one reason our prescription drug prices and hospital charges are higher than other countries, many of whom engage in centralized price negotiations.[108] We leave price negotiations up to individual health insurance plans to negotiate with hospitals, physicians and pharmaceutical companies, missing out on the benefits of a central body negotiating bulk discounts.[109] Thus, we often wind up paying more.

Our complex and fragmented medical structure results in higher administrative overhead too. In fact, we spent $812 billion in administrative costs in 2017, perhaps comprising as much as 30

---

[107] Sarah Kliff and Soo Oh, "America's health care prices are out of control. These 11 charts prove it." *Vox.com* May 10, 2018 https://www.vox.com/a/health-prices
[108] Dana Sarnak, David Squires and Shawn Bishop. "Paying for Prescription Drugs Around the World: Why is the US the Outlier?" *The Commonwealth Fund*, October 2017 https://www.commonwealthfund.org/publications/issue-briefs/2017/oct/paying-prescription-drugs-around-world-why-us-outlier
[109] https://www.vox.com/a/health-prices

percent of total healthcare spending.[110] [111] That is $600 billion more than Canada spends, which also has four times lower per capita administrative costs.[112]

Writing in the Harvard Business Review, Dr. Robert Kocher, formerly of the McKinsey Global Institute, noted that "for every doctor (in the U.S.), only 6 of the 16 non-doctor workers have clinical roles, including registered nurses, allied health professionals, aides, care coordinators, and medical assistants. Surprisingly, 10 of the 16 non-doctor workers are purely administrative and management staff, receptionists and information clerks, and office clerks. The problem with all of the non-doctor labor is that most of it is not primarily associated with delivering better patient outcomes or lowering costs."[113]

Our fragmented, multi-payer system — with its different private insurance programs, government payors at the federal, state and

---

[110] Zachary Henderson, "A study reveals the US could save $600 in administrative costs by switching to a single-payer, Medicare for all System," Business insider, January 8, 2020 https://www.businessinsider.com/single-payer-system-could-save-us-massive-administrative-costs-2020-1

[111] Joshua Gottlieb and Mark Shepard, "How Large a Burden are Administrative Costs in Health Care? *Econofact 2020* https://econofact.org/how-large-a-burden-are-administrative-costs-in-health-care

[112] Zachary Henderson, "A study reveals the US could save $600 in administrative costs by switching to a single-payer, *Medicare for all System*," Business insider, January 8, 2020 https://www.businessinsider.com/single-payer-system-could-save-us-massive-administrative-costs-2020-1

[113] Robert Kocher, "The Downside of Health Care Growth", Harvard Business Review, Sept. 23,2013. https://hbr.org/2013/09/the-downside-of-health-care-job-growth

local level, etc. — and all the complex billing arrangements that exist are a major reason for the high administrative costs.[114] An estimated $265 billion annually is wasted due to administrative complexity alone. This helps to explain at least partially why healthcare has become so expensive for patients.

Another major driver of healthcare costs in states like California is hospital consolidation, according to state attorney general Xavier Becerra. The state is engaged in a lawsuit with a hospital chain, Sutter Heath, which it alleges through multiple mergers and acquisitions has essentially became a monopoly, driving up healthcare prices for Californians. In a "60 Minutes" report in December 2020, Becerra said Sutter was "gobbling up hospitals…gobbling up physicians. They were just munching away, getting bigger and bigger. The hospital chain," Becerra said, "got big enough that it could use its market power to dominate, to dictate. It was abusing its power." Sutter Health has now 24 hospitals, 12,000 physicians and several specialty centers.[115]

---

[114] Joshua Gottlieb and Mark Shepard, "How Large a Burden are Administrative Costs in Health Care? *Econofact 2020* https://econofact.org/how-large-a-burden-are-administrative-costs-in-health-care

[115] Lesley Stahl, "How a hospital system grew to gain market power and drove up healthcare costs," *CBSnews.com*, 60 Minutes, December 13, 2020. https://www.cbsnews.com/news/california-sutter-health-hospital-chain-high-prices-lawsuit-60-minutes-2020-12-13/

By cornering the market on healthcare, California's lawsuit says, Sutter was able to "jack up prices." Example: The costs for care of a premature baby in Northern California is about $605,000 compared to about $343,000 in Southern California. Overall, inpatient care is 70 percent higher in Northern versus Southern California. Becerra said rising healthcare prices are due to "domination of the market."[116]

Glenn Melnick, a healthcare economist at the University of Southern California who consulted on the lawsuit, said, "They (Sutter) really pioneered this model of reducing competition to raise prices. They were the first one to do it." The problem, he said, is that Sutter raised prices without improving quality, value, or service. Furthermore, he said their practices have enabled Sutter's competitors to raise their prices too. Hillary Ronen, who sits on San Francisco's city and county board of supervisors, says, "It's outrageous…Sutter won't allow us to see how much they charge for their services. It's unbelievable. And so we can't comparison shop. And they keep naming their price, and I'm handcuffed to do anything about it."[117]

Ronen said that Sutter, because of its not-for-profit status has also avoided paying tens of millions of dollars a year in property taxes.

---

[116] Stahl, 60 Minutes. *CBSnews.com.*
[117] Stahl, 60 Minutes. *CBSnews.com.*

Elizabeth Mitchell CEO of Pacific Business Group on Health, said that while other industries have used their size to lower costs, "the opposite has been true in healthcare. They merge and they use their market leverage to increase prices." This is happening, by the way, in hospitals all over the county, like Maine, Texas, etc. "The largest health systems are buying up everything," Mitchell said. She has looked at the data and says hospital pricing is the largest driver of healthcare cost increases. "It's hospital prices. And they're not providing more services. And the quality isn't increasing. They are just charging more for the same thing. It is just the prices because they can."[118]

Sutter has tentatively agreed to a settlement in which it will pay $575 million, agree to stop preventing patients from accessing less expensive hospitals, and admit no wrongdoing. Becerra sees this as a potential "game changer" for hundreds of thousands of Californians and possibly millions of Americans, where other hospital systems may be acting similarly.[119]

Needless to say, high prices, waste and greed are at issue here. Add to this that a study published in JAMA showed that $1 out of every $4 spent (or between $760 billion and $935 billion) is wasted on healthcare as a whole every year, and we can begin to

---
[118] Stahl, 60 Minutes. *CBSnews.com.*
[119] Stahl, 60 Minutes. *CBSnews.com.*

understand how pervasive and systemic the issue is.[120] And when we consider that one in four U.S. consumers has delayed treatment for a serious illness due to rising medical costs and 67 percent of all bankruptcies in the U.S. are due to exorbitant healthcare costs (per a 2019 study), we realize that healthcare expenditures are indeed spiraling out of control.[121] Reform becomes a must.

Unfortunately, we don't even benefit from all this spending. According to research from the Commonwealth Fund, the U.S. ranks last in life expectancy among similar high-income countries, but first in suicides.[122] We have the highest rate of avoidable deaths for conditions like heart disease, diabetes, or cancer, and the highest chronic disease burden (such as asthma, high blood pressure, and heart disease).

The awful advent of the novel coronavirus should provoke a hard look at our inefficient and needlessly complicated system – and serious ideas for reforming it. Ideally, we want a system that will

---

[120] Bruce D. Broussard, "Humana study reveals $265 billion wasted on health care each year in the US," *CNBC.com*, October 7, 2019 https://www.cnbc.com/2019/10/07/study-reveals-265-billion-wasted-on-health-care-each-year-in-us.html

[121] Zachary Henderson, "A study reveals the US could save $600 in administrative costs by switching to a single-payer, Medicare for all System," *Business Insider*, January 8, 2020 https://www.businessinsider.com/single-payer-system-could-save-us-massive-administrative-costs-2020-1

[122] Roosa Tikkanen & Melinda Abrams, "U.S. Health Care from a Global Perspective, 2019: Higher Spending, Worse Outcomes?" *The Commonwealth Fund*, January 30, 2020 https://www.commonwealthfund.org/publications/issue-briefs/2020/jan/us-health-care-global-perspective-2019

take care of all of us, including those who have had COVID or post-COVID symptoms over the long haul. America's current fee-for-service model, which bills patients for every line item and every procedure, incentivizes physicians to do more and bill more. We need a system that prioritizes health outcomes over volume.

What can we do? In both his book and a subsequent conversation with me, Spellberg embraced the idea of a single-payer system (the type where the government pays private and county hospitals to deliver care) with an optional private insurance buy-in.[123]

"Single-payer systems throughout the world deliver better outcomes at much lower cost than private multi-payer systems do," he said. "That is an objective reality." The system would include healthcare for all via a public health plan, funded by central federal taxes collected from everyone. Private insurance options would exist for those who wish to purchase them, but these individuals would still contribute funds to the public plan. Australia and New Zealand are two countries that operate this way; costs are much lower, the systems perform very well, and average life expectancies are longer.

Under this model, businesses would no longer be burdened with

---

[123] Brad Spellberg. *Broken, Bankrupt and Dying*. Lioncrest Publishing 2020.

paying for their employees' healthcare, enabling them to be more competitive in the global marketplace. (U.S. companies spend more than $620 billion on such care annually.)[124] Public and private insurance companies would be able to coexist and compete against one another. In Canada, 25 million people have purchased additional private insurance, despite most of their 37.5 million citizens being insured by the government.[125]

Administrative costs would be drastically reduced with a simplified single-payer system (cost savings estimates range between $200 billion and $500 billion), and care would improve as the financial incentives become more aligned with quality rather than quantity.[126] [127] Pharmaceutical drug prices would be negotiated downward and out-of-pocket expenses minimized. Price transparency would actually exist.

Americans want options. We want access to affordable,

---

[124] Timothy Denney, Healthcare costs are harming U.S. Competitiveness, International Policy Digest, June 17, 2019, https://intpolicydigest.org/2019/06/17/healthcare-costs-are-harming-u-s-competitiveness/
[125] "How Many Americans are Uninsured (2020)," *PolicyAdvice.net*, November 22, 2020, https://policyadvice.net/insurance/insights/how-many-uninsured-americans/
[126] William Shrank, Teresa Rogstad, Natasha Parekh, "Waste in the US Health Care System Estimated Costs and Potential for Savings," *JAMA Network*, October 7, 2019 https://jamanetwork.com/journals/jama/article-abstract/2752664
[127] Steffie Woolhandler, MD, MPH and David Himmelstein, MD, "Single-Payer Reform: The only way to Fulfill the President's Pledge of More Coverage, Better Benefits, and Lower Costs," *Annals of Internal Medicine*, February 21, 2017 https://mfprac.com/web2020/07literature/literature/Health_Costs/SinglePayer_Woolhandler1.pdf

streamlined healthcare. And in the midst of a pandemic, we certainly want universal coverage that does not deny those with pre-existing conditions.

Spellberg notes that change in the U.S. is not a problem of knowledge, but a "problem of will and politics." In this case, though, even two-fifths of Republicans have indicated that they would favor single-payer reform.[128] And we know it can be done, because other countries are already doing it. It is time for each of us to demand change, so that all of us have access to healthcare while retaining our tried-and-true American value of free choice.

A big first step is to stop treating a single-payer plan as a hostile force, but rather a way to take care of our own. And the next step, of course, is to insist that healthcare reform be placed front and center of the national agenda.

---

[128] Steffie Woolhandler, MD, MPH and David Himmelstein, MD, "Single-Payer Reform: The only way to Fulfill the President's Pledge of More Coverage, Better Benefits, and Lower Costs," *Annals of Internal Medicine*, February 21, 2017 https://mfprac.com/web2020/07literature/literature/Health_Costs/SinglePayer_Woolhandler1.pdf

Recently, a screening ultrasound revealed two suspicious nodules in my neck, leading my doctors to worry that my cancer might have returned after 30 years. I consulted a very experienced oncologist, who suggested a complete neck dissection, potentially radiation treatment again, and a chest CT scan now to look for metastases — yet he agreed that none of it would improve the chances of survival. Two other doctors advocated for watchful waiting, which is where I'm headed.

This possible recurrence may or may not have something to do with the radiation treatment I received in 1987. Regardless, I didn't know any better at the time. Doesn't that describe a majority of us, in most critical medical situations?

That has to change. Some key moves toward transparency within the power corridors of medicine and industry will go a long way. Our hospitals and specialty organizations can help reduce overtesting by uncoupling physician pay and test ordering. They can move away from the fee-for-service model and toward value-based care, where providers are reimbursed for services that lead to better health outcomes. They can develop uniform clinical practice guidelines, so practitioners have clear indications of when NOT to test. And they can seek medical tort reform to reduce the pressure physicians feel to test more and practice defensive medicine.

An American Medical Association (AMA) 2016 Benchmark Survey showed that one-third of all physicians had been sued during their time practicing.[129] In certain specialties, that risk runs as high as 63 percent. The pressure not to miss something is real, and it is costly.

Regulatory agencies can impose strict limitations on medical-industry relationships to prevent financial conflicts of interest and uphold the integrity of our scientific research. Drug manufacturers should not be permitted to ghostwrite studies under the guise of science, nor to pay physician experts to promote off-label use of drugs for medical conditions for which they have not been proven to work.

I also second several of the recommendations made by Dr. Angell: Industry should not be allowed to sponsor its own clinical trials. Big Pharma should not be funding physicians' medical education or sponsoring our national symposiums. Direct-to-consumer advertising/sales pitches by industry should be eliminated to

---

[129] Jose Guardado, "Medical Liability Claim Frequency Among U.S. Physicians" *AMA Economic and Health Policy Research*, December 2017 https://www.ama-assn.org/sites/ama-assn.org/files/corp/media-browser/public/government/advocacy/policy-research-perspective-medical-liability-claim-frequency.pdf

reduce patients' demand for drugs and testing.[130]

We need to establish an agency to set maximum allowable prescription drug prices (or at least negotiate with drugmakers over price), cap drug price increases, and approve only cost-effective drugs that are proven to be clinically better than existing ones. The agency would restrict the duration of patent protection for medications to around 7 to 10 years after a drug's first entry, incentivize and scale contracts for American-made generics, and eliminate "pay-for-delay" schemes, where brand-name drug companies pay generic manufacturers to delay their drug's entry to market. [131]

We also need a plan to finance medical education: graduating from medical school and being $200,000 to $300,000 in debt can be a powerful inducement to say "yes" when Big Pharma and the device industry come calling.

As a society, let's mandate healthcare for all. Everyone deserves access. I've seen too many people leave our emergency departments with serious illness — or not seek care at all because they could not afford that care. Not only is care a moral

---
[130] Marcia Angell, MD, The Truth About the Drug Companies. *Random House Books*, Aug 9, 2005.
[131] Vincent Rajkumar, "The high cost of prescriptions drugs; causes and solutions," *Nature*, June 23, 2020 https://www.nature.com/articles/s41408-020-0338-x#ref-CR12

imperative, but our country will function better if people are healthy, contributing members of society.

As physicians, we need to do the lion's share of the work. We need to choose very wisely when making recommendations for our patients. We need to read primarily non-industry funded research, ensure our decisions are in our patients' best interests (or at least not conflicted), and think through and discuss the risks versus benefits with our patients so they can make informed decisions. And sometimes we need to consider recommending the option of doing nothing. If collectively we can reduce "unnecessary services" by half the Institute of Medicine estimates it will reduce health care expenditures by $105 billion every year.[132] We can further shrink costs by prescribing generic drugs first, and by only prescribing branded, more expensive "me too" medicines if they demonstrate improved efficacy. This may seem obvious, but Big Pharma will always push hard in the other direction.

And although this may seem self-evident, it bears saying out loud: Let's beef up preventive care. This is as opposed to concentrating on emergent, expensive, procedure-oriented care. We should invest in primary care, in social services, public health clinics,

---

[132] Heather Lyu, "Overtreatment in the United States", PLoS One. 2017 https://www.ncbi.nlm.nih.gov/pmc/articles/PMC5587107/#!po=55.8824/

home visits and the like. Some 40% of all emergency department visits are non-urgent.[133] This is some of the most expensive care there is. In fact, an estimated $18 billion could be saved annually if these patients were seen at primary care facilities instead of emergency departments.[134] COVID-19 has made the underinvestment and inadequacies of our public health system glaringly apparent.[135] Let's build up this infrastructure and workforce to promote health services to all people in all communities, especially our more vulnerable.

My own journey with disease has led me to another discovery. With all of my experience and ability to ask the right questions, I still find it nearly impossible to learn my surgeon's success rate, rate of complications, infection, readmission and re-operation. That's the kind of information hospitals don't make available. Let's change that too.

Politicians have been talking about it for so long that it seems almost blasé to say it, but healthcare needs to be affordable. Affordable or not, though, right now it is nearly impossible to

---

[133] CDC National Center for Health Statistics, *CDC*, https://www.cdc.gov/nchs/fastats/emergency-department.htm
[134] Bill Fay, "Emergency Rooms vs Urgent Care Centers," *Debt.org*, https://www.debt.org/medical/emergency-room-urgent-care-costs/
[135] Brian Dixon, et al. "Deficient Response to COVID-19 Makes the Case for Evolving the Public Health System, *American Journal of Preventive Medicine* August 26, 2020 https://www.ajpmonline.org/article/S0749-3797(20)30369-X/fulltext

determine the cost of a hospitalization ahead of time. Have you ever purchased a car without knowing the price? Without being able to compare prices easily, market forces don't work to restrain costs. We need price transparency with mandated price disclosures, we need to eliminate surprise billing (whereby patients have to pay out-of-network charges of which they were not aware), we need to rein in high-insurance deductibles, premiums, copayments, etc., and we need to put an end to hospital price gouging that leaves patients on the hook for astronomical bills that they cannot pay.[136] Approximately, one in five Americans has serious medical debt.[137]

To put it plain, we're broken. We have a morass of government programs, insurance companies, healthcare providers, hospitals, outpatient surgery centers, and clinics providing expensive and uncoordinated care. The system needs to be streamlined for everyone: patients, providers, and payors. Our current mess is responsible for physician/practitioner burnout, endless scheduling and billing frustrations, patient frustrations, wasted money, and wasted time.

---

[136] Ge Bai and Gerard Anderson, "Extreme Markup: The fifty US Hospitals with the Highest Charge-To-Cost Ratios," *Health Affairs*, June 2015.
https://pnhp.org/news/for-profit-hospitals-lead-the-way-in-price-gouging/
[137] Chris Coffey, "Nearly 1 in 5 Americans Has Crippling Medical Debt," *NBC Chicago*, March 12 2018, https://www.nbcchicago.com/news/local/1-in-5-americans-has-crippling-medical-debt/163416/

Affordable, transparent, quality care with better health outcomes across the board – this is what Americans deserve and should expect. I believe that a single-payer system with a vibrant, independent private-insurer market could go a long way toward solving many of these issues.

This not the time for incrementalism. With the new President-elect, we have an opportunity to dramatically reframe the conversation around our healthcare system. In doing so, the administration could save more lives than we doctors can do in our entire lifetimes.

None of this is easy, as I've experienced first-hand. In my own case, I'm extremely grateful for the care I've received over the last 30 years, for having some excellent role models, and for being alive. I have worked with and among many wonderful physicians, and I can attest that their jobs are difficult and challenging. Some pharmaceutical and medical-device companies have made significant advances in healthcare, too. But, now is the time to think very seriously about our next steps. Now is the time to put the emphasis on quality, patient-first care.

And some already do. My two personal oncology physicians were the ones who advised a conservative strategy of monitoring those nodules in my neck, which could prove to be benign. As they explained it to me, they believe the harm of surgically removing them, with all of the potential complications, far outweighs the benefit. I'm ever appreciative of their reflection, care and honesty. I believe they deeply honored their Hippocratic Oath: First, do no harm.

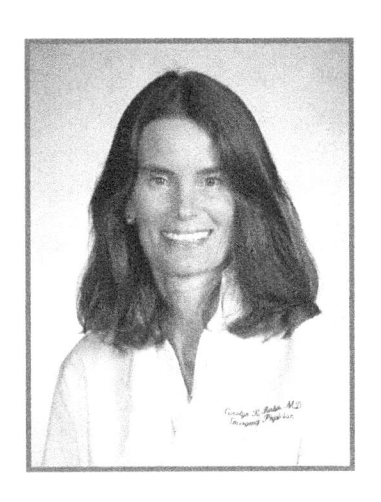

Carolyn Barber, M.D., earned her B.A. from Princeton University, did her medical training at Johns Hopkins School of Medicine and completed her residency at Stanford University Medical Center. An emergency department physician for 25 years, she is also cofounder of a homeless work program in San Diego, Wheels of Change, which has received CNN's 2020 "Champion for Change" award.

Dr. Barber is a nationally published author. Her writings on COVID-19 related issues and treatments have appeared in Fortune, Scientific American, the New York Daily News, the San Diego Union Tribune, and numerous other news outlets. They can be found on her website: www.carolynbarbermd.com.

Made in United States
Orlando, FL
04 February 2024